Katie-Jane Crosbie

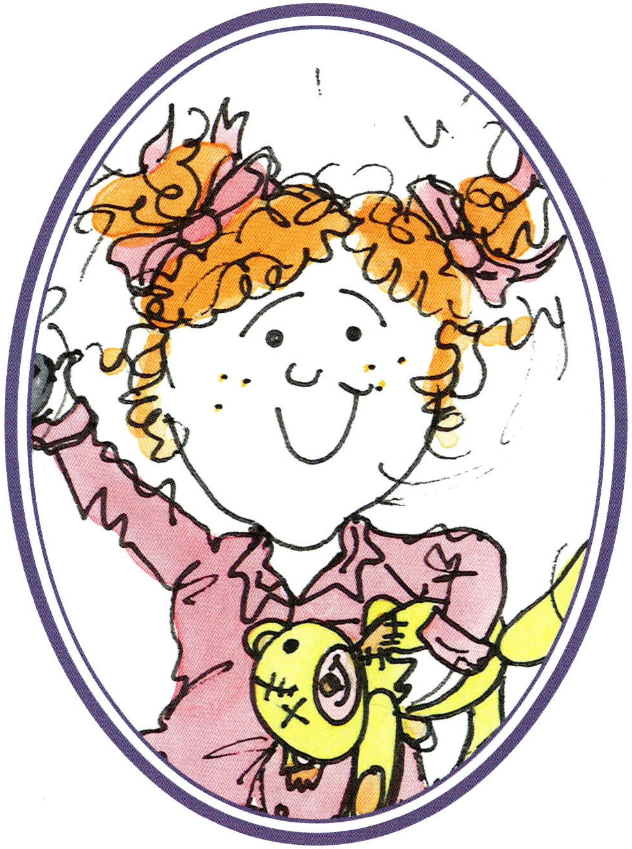

Lizzie's Best Sleep Ever!

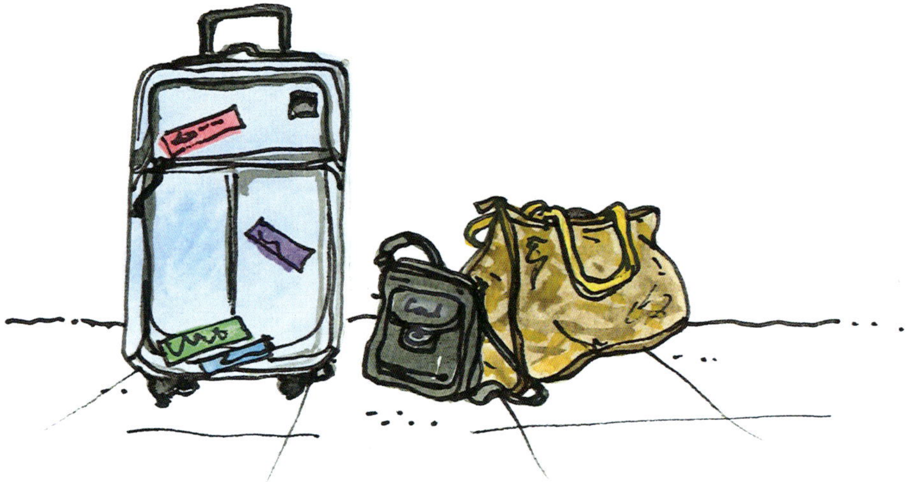

ISBN 978 1 5272 9368 7
First published in Great Britain in 2021.
This edition published in 2021 in Liverpool, U.K.

This is Lizzie. Lizzie is always tired.

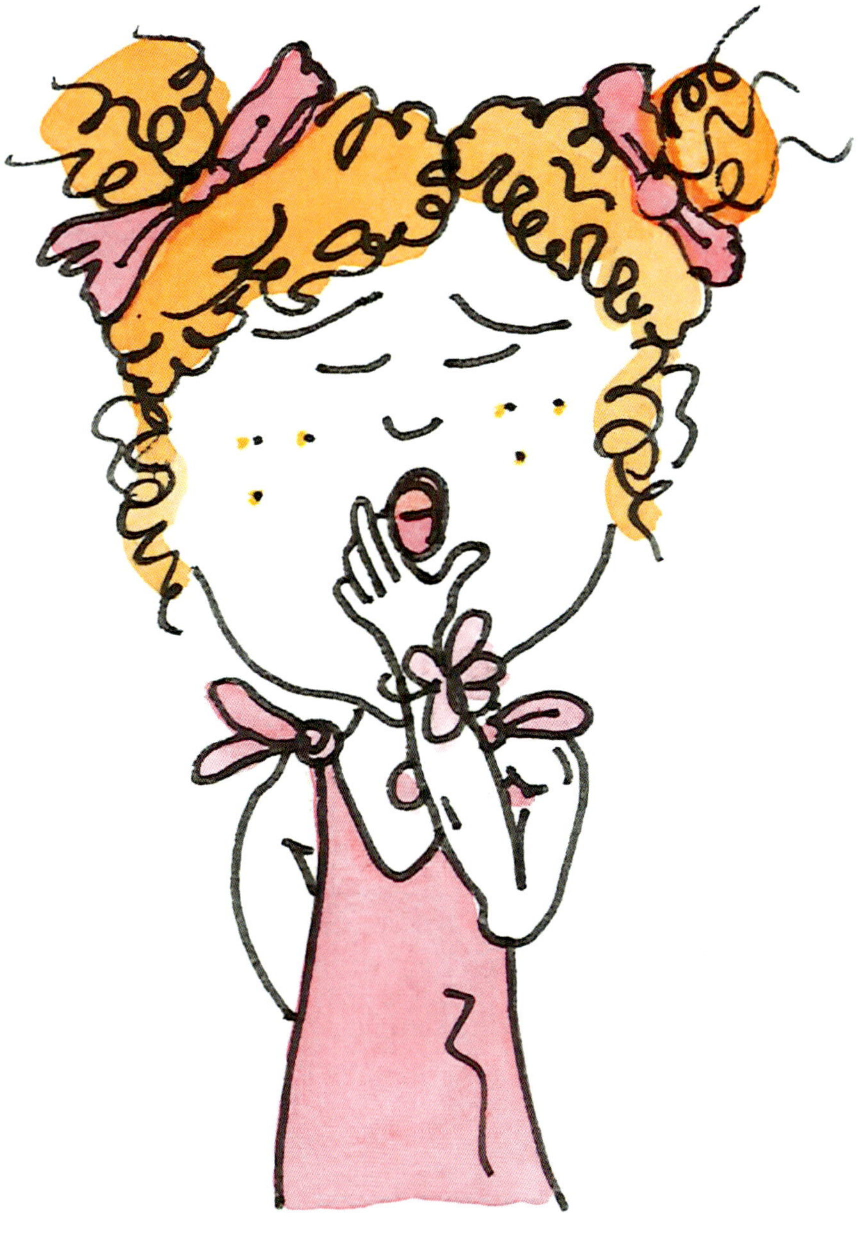

She feels grumpy all day and never finishes her meals.

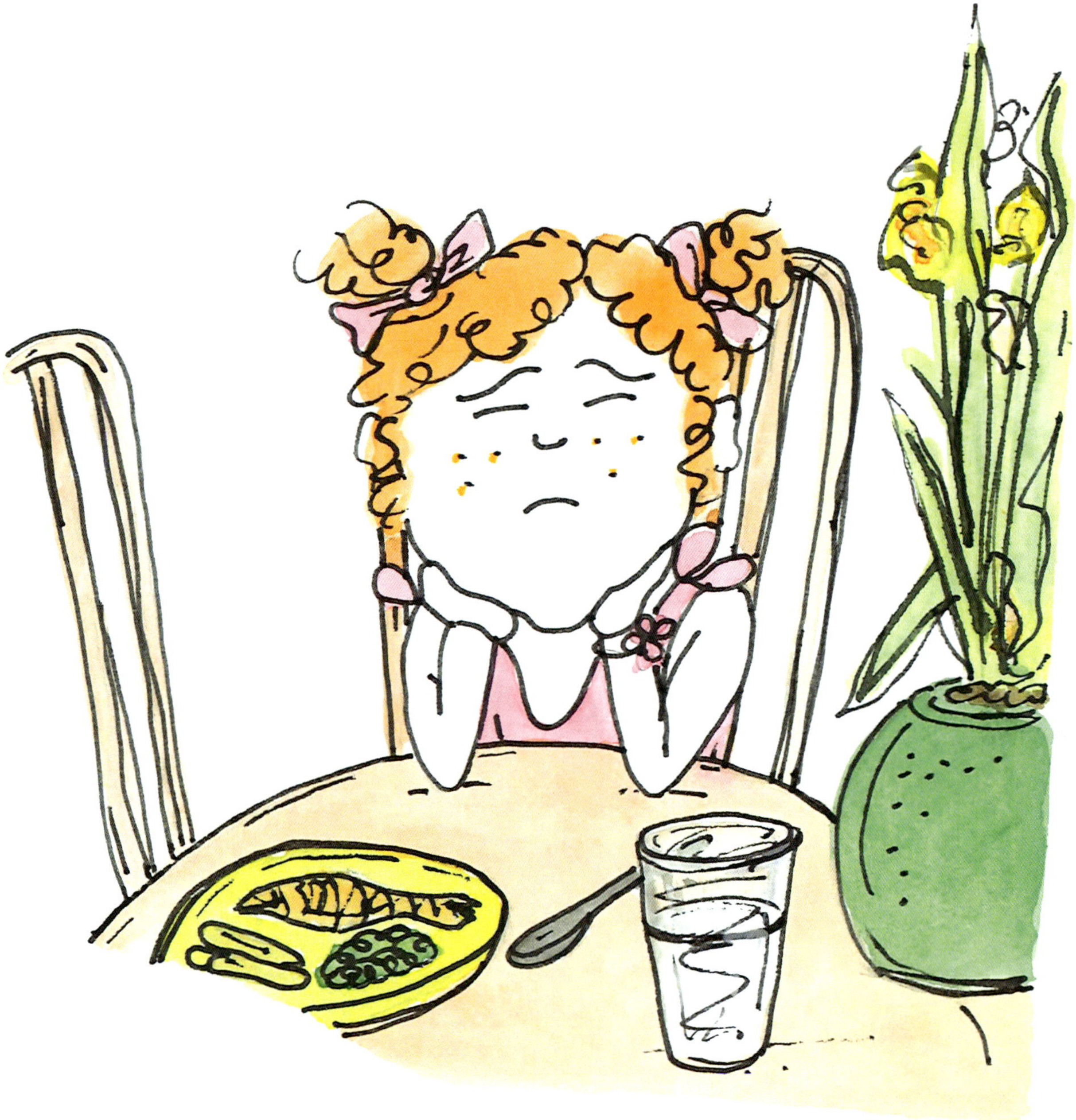

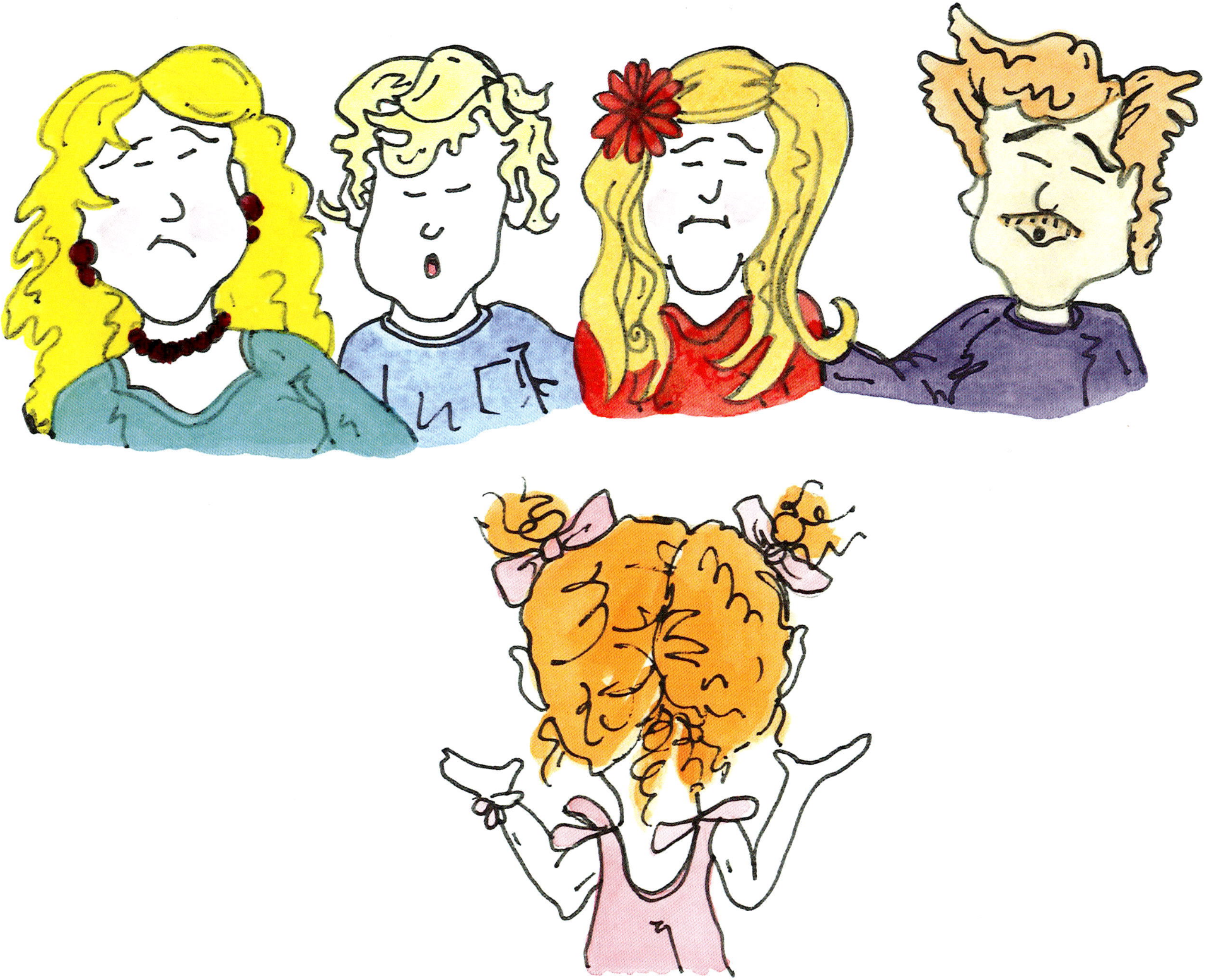

All of her family are VERY tired too!

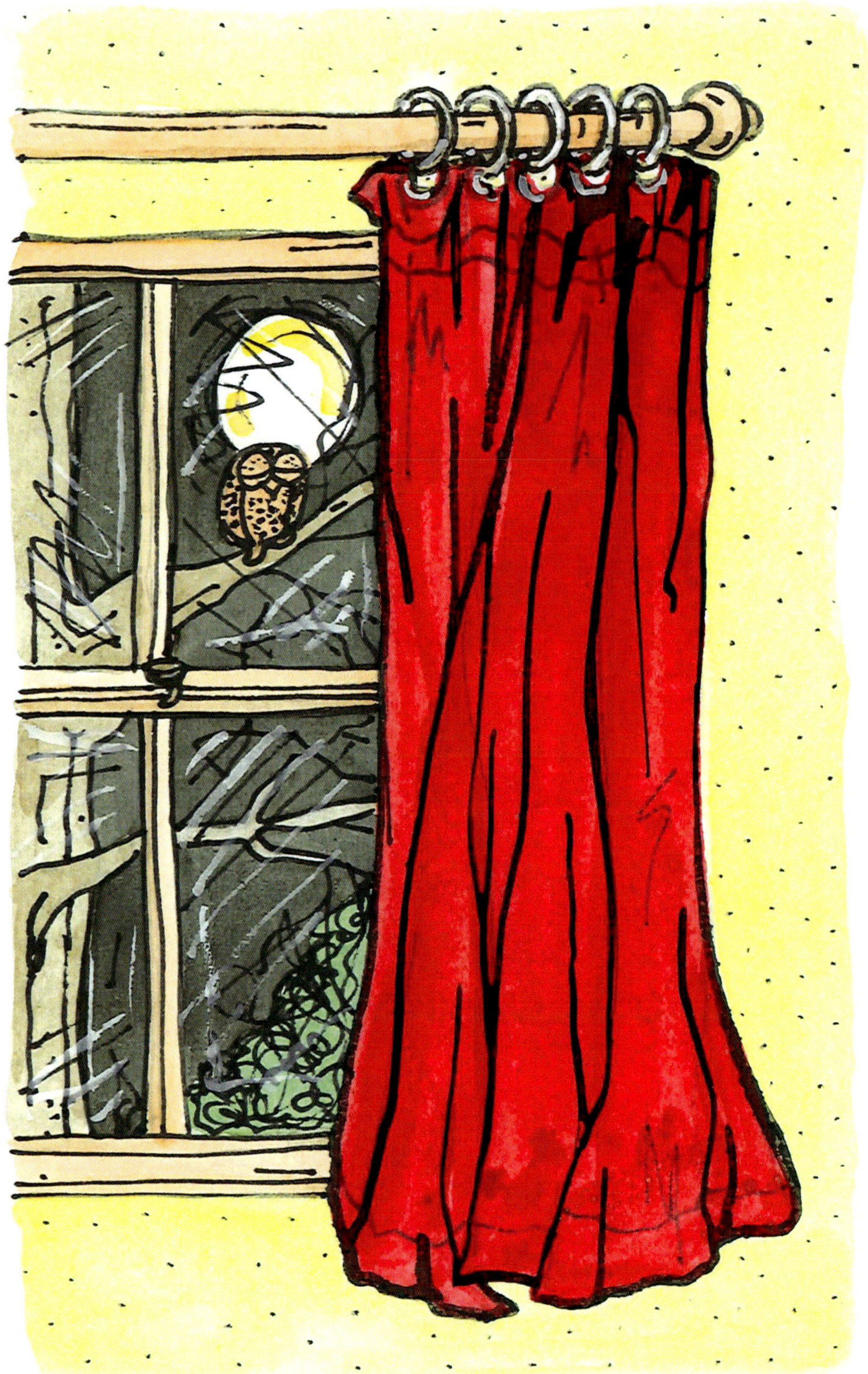

Why?

Lizzie keeps them up all night,
so every time she wakes they try to....

....give her another Teddy bear
to sleep with....

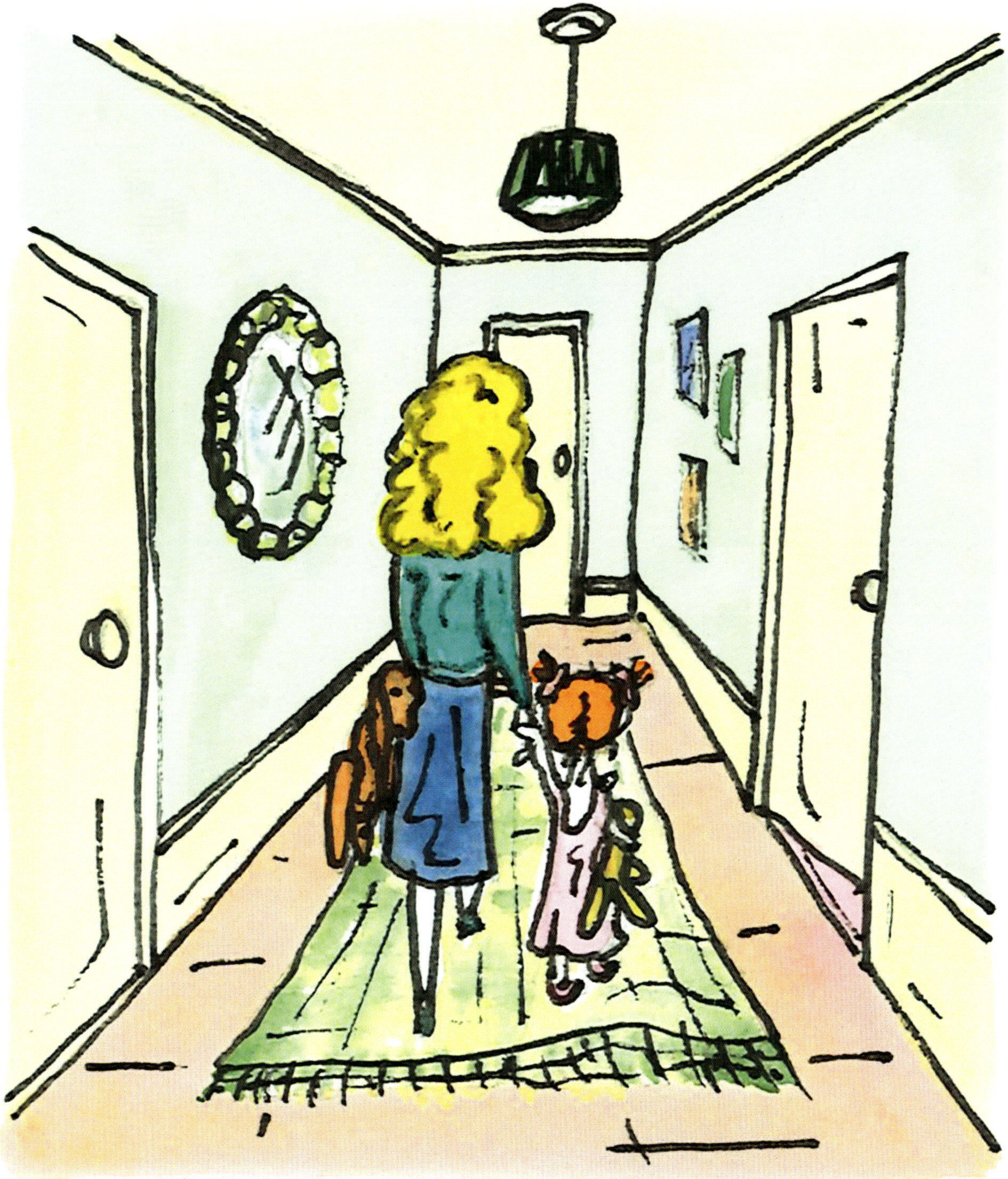

....take her back to bed -

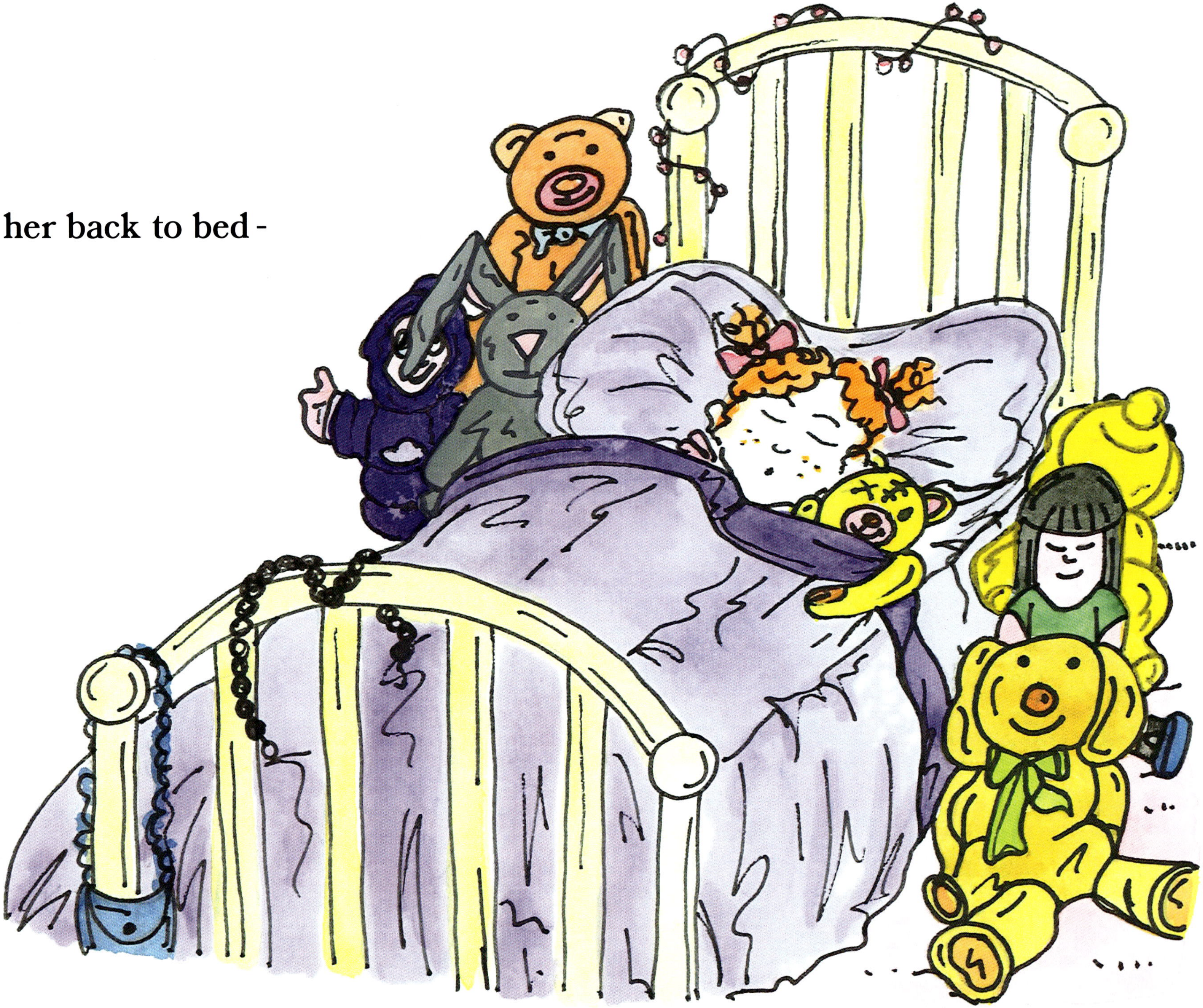

Make her a drink and rock her to sleep on their knee!

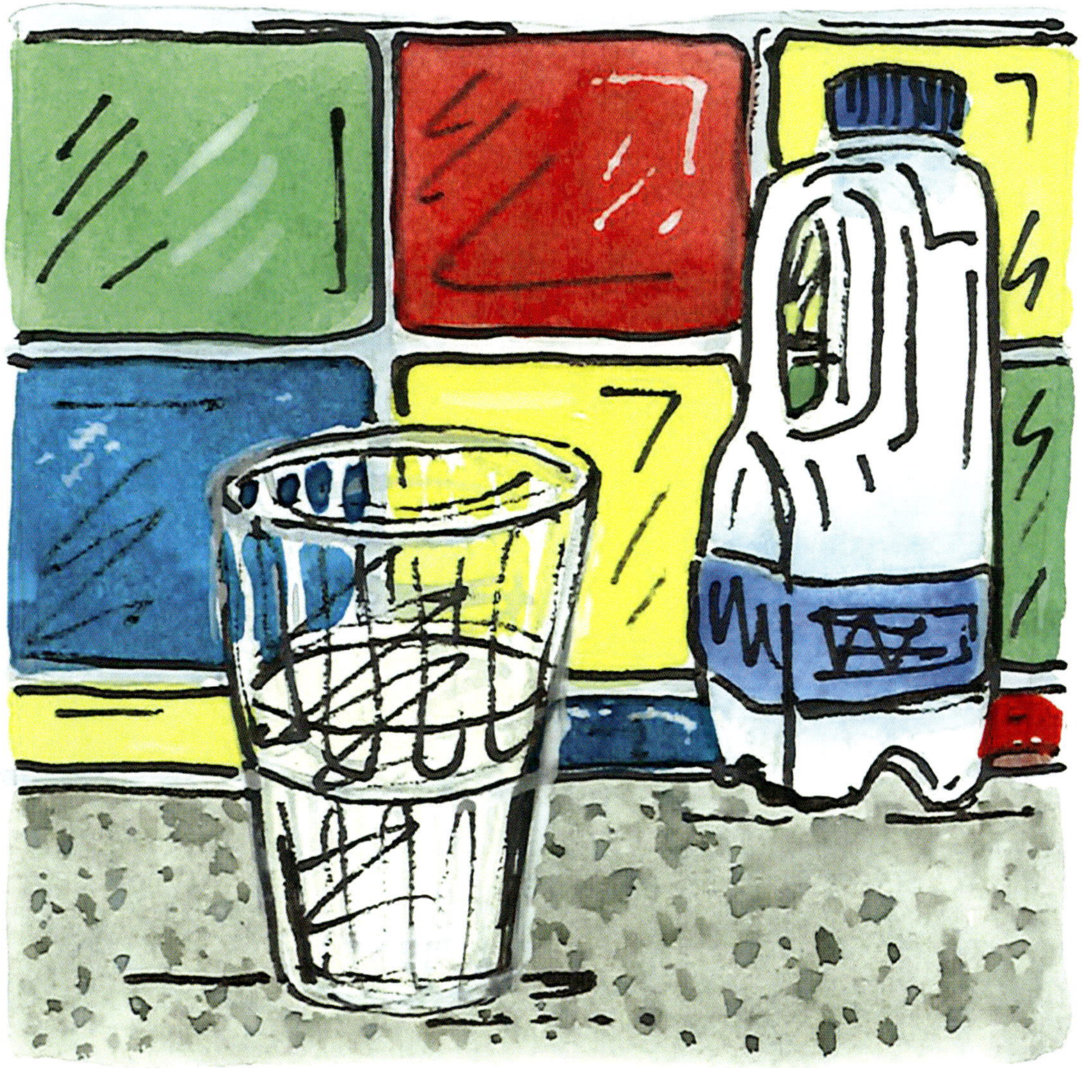

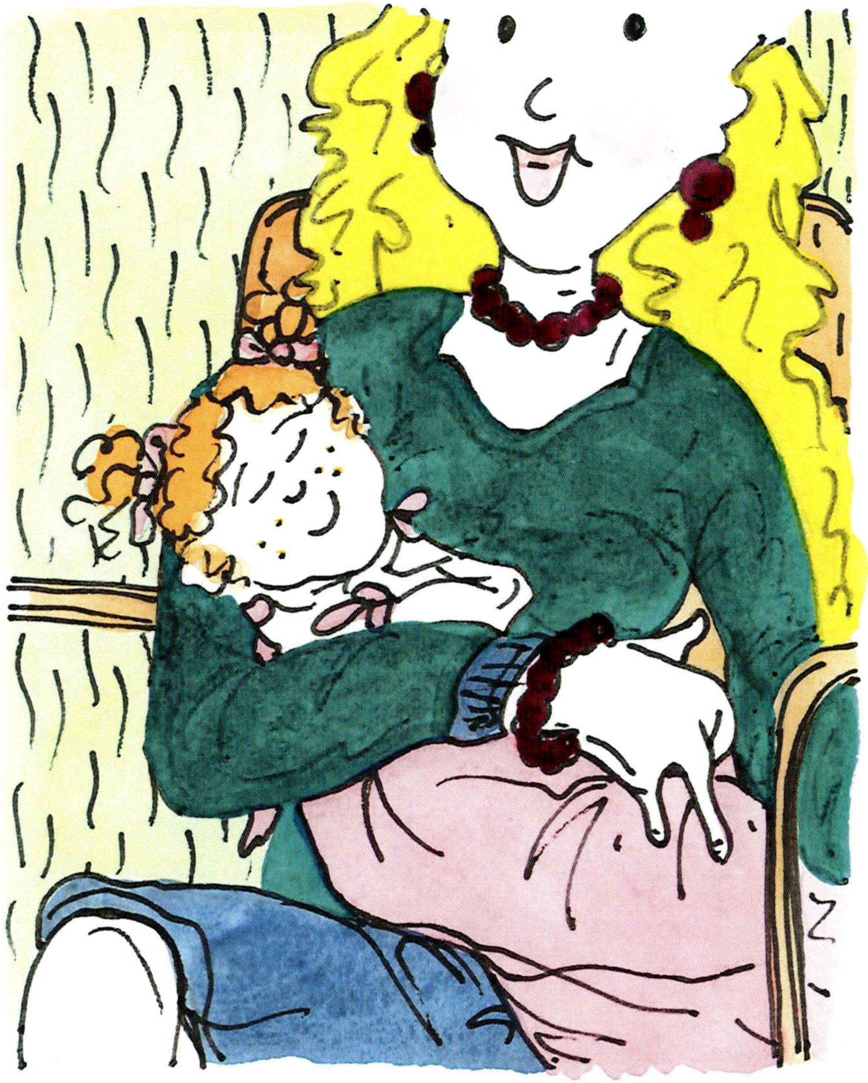

No matter how many times they get Lizzie to fall back asleep, she ALWAYS wakes a few hours later!

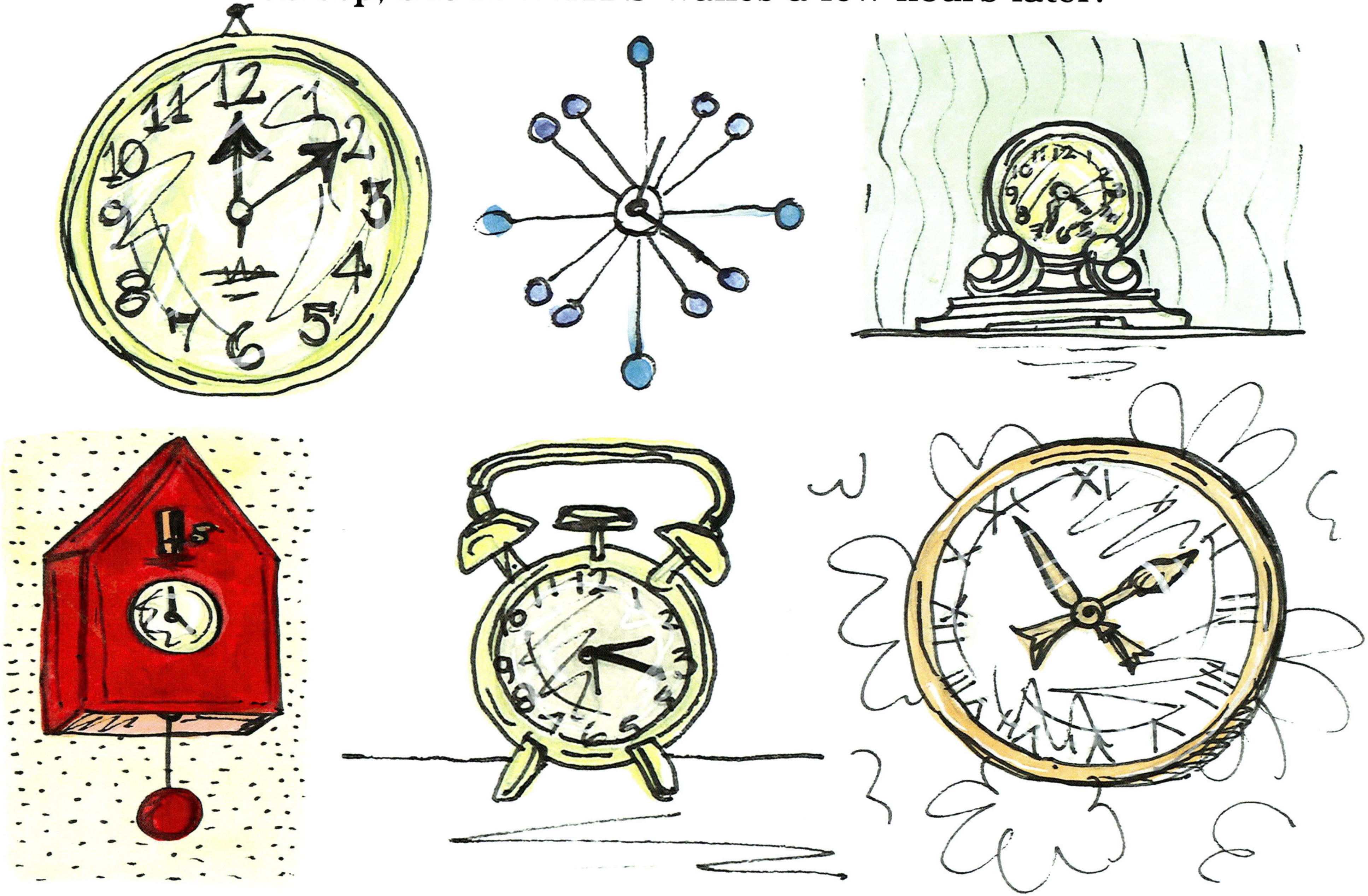

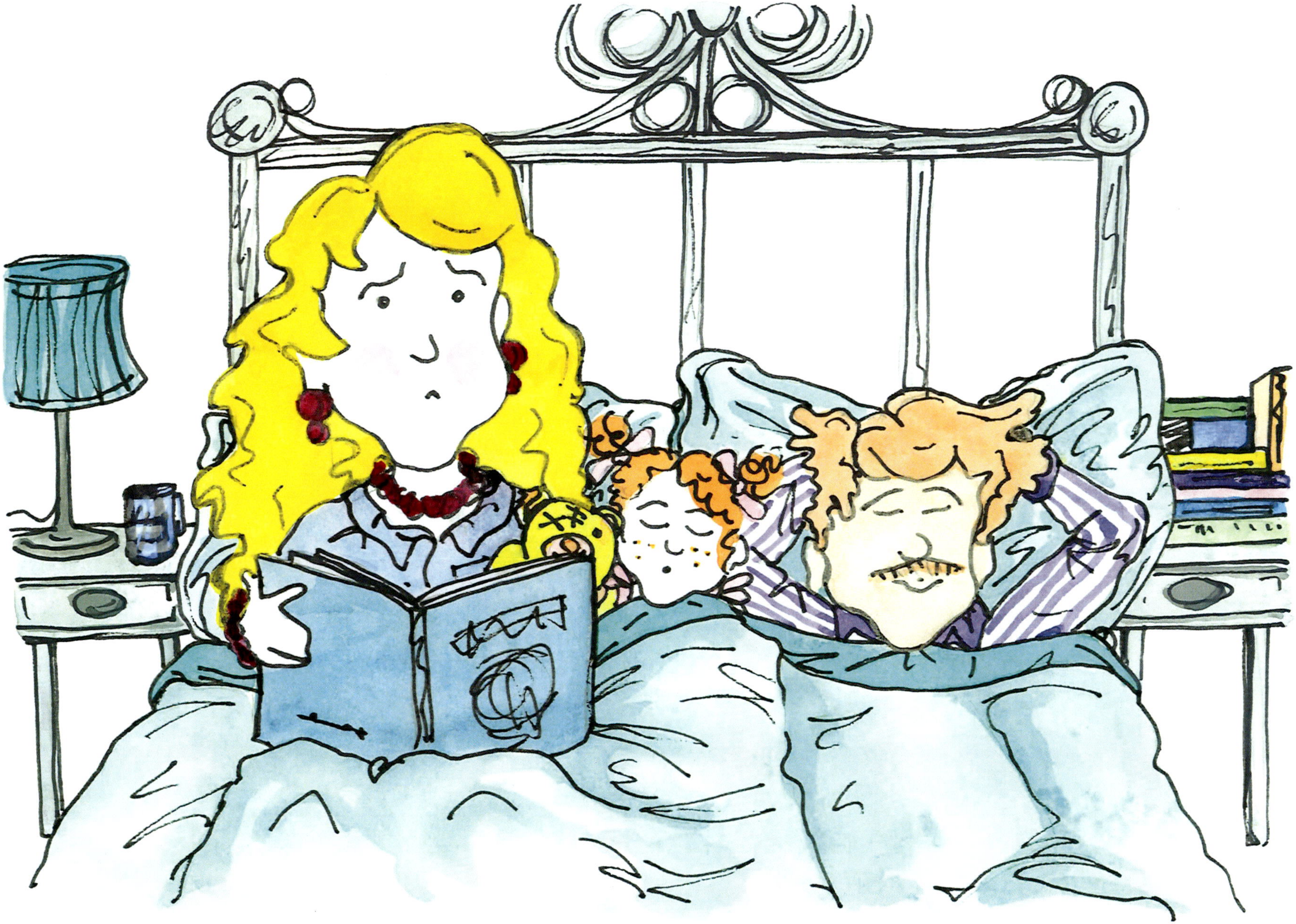

After her parents have tried everything to get her back to sleep in her own bed - guess what? Lizzie always ends up sleeping in their bed!

Lizzie's parents phoned a lovely lady called Katie-Jane - but you can call her KJ!

Everyone else calls her The International Baby Whisperer.

Lizzie thought that was a very silly name, but KJ teaches children how to sleep and be rested.

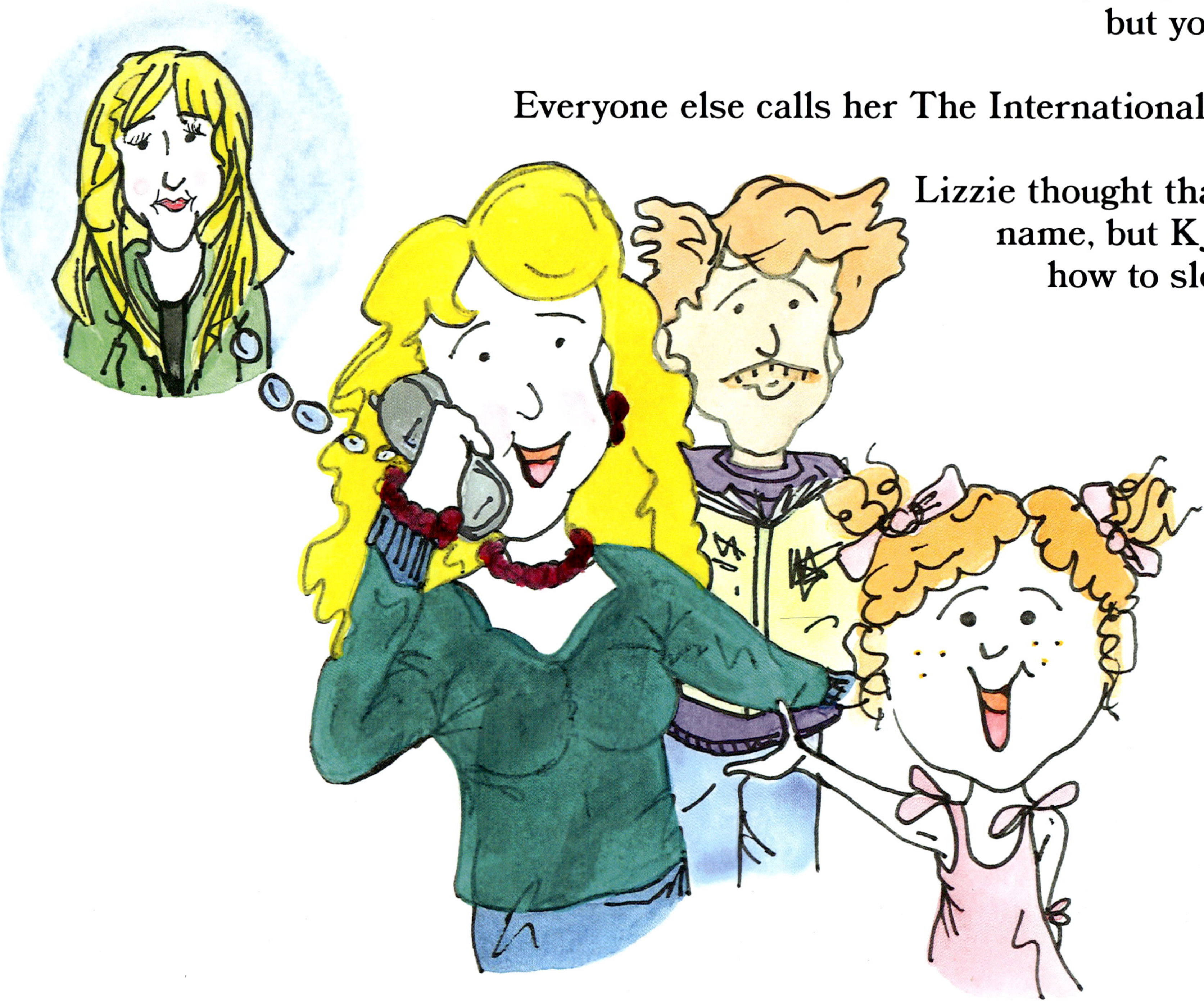

When KJ came to visit Lizzie's home, she talked about how important sleep is for all the family.

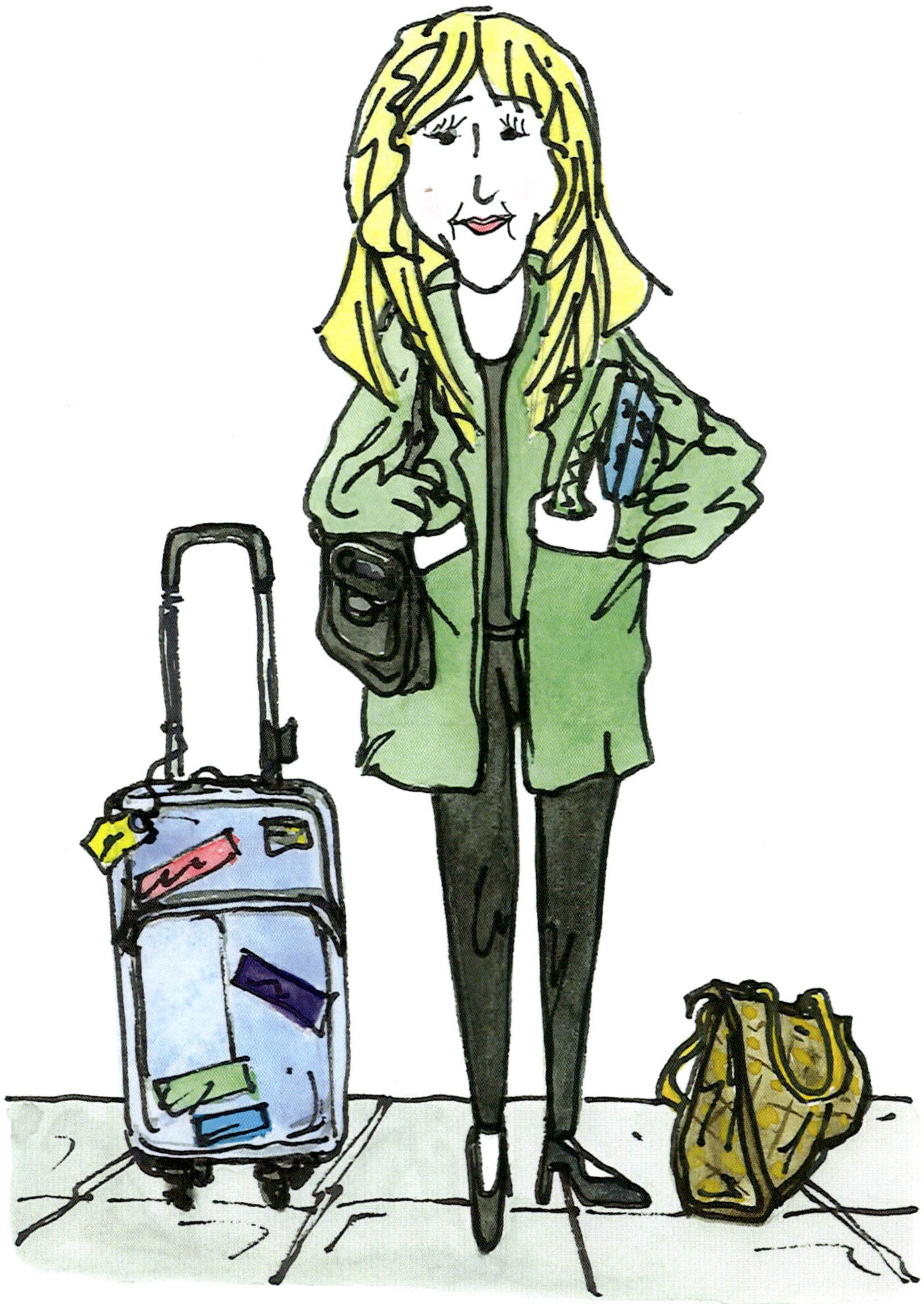

It is important children do not watch television before bedtime.
They may stay very wide awake and excited.

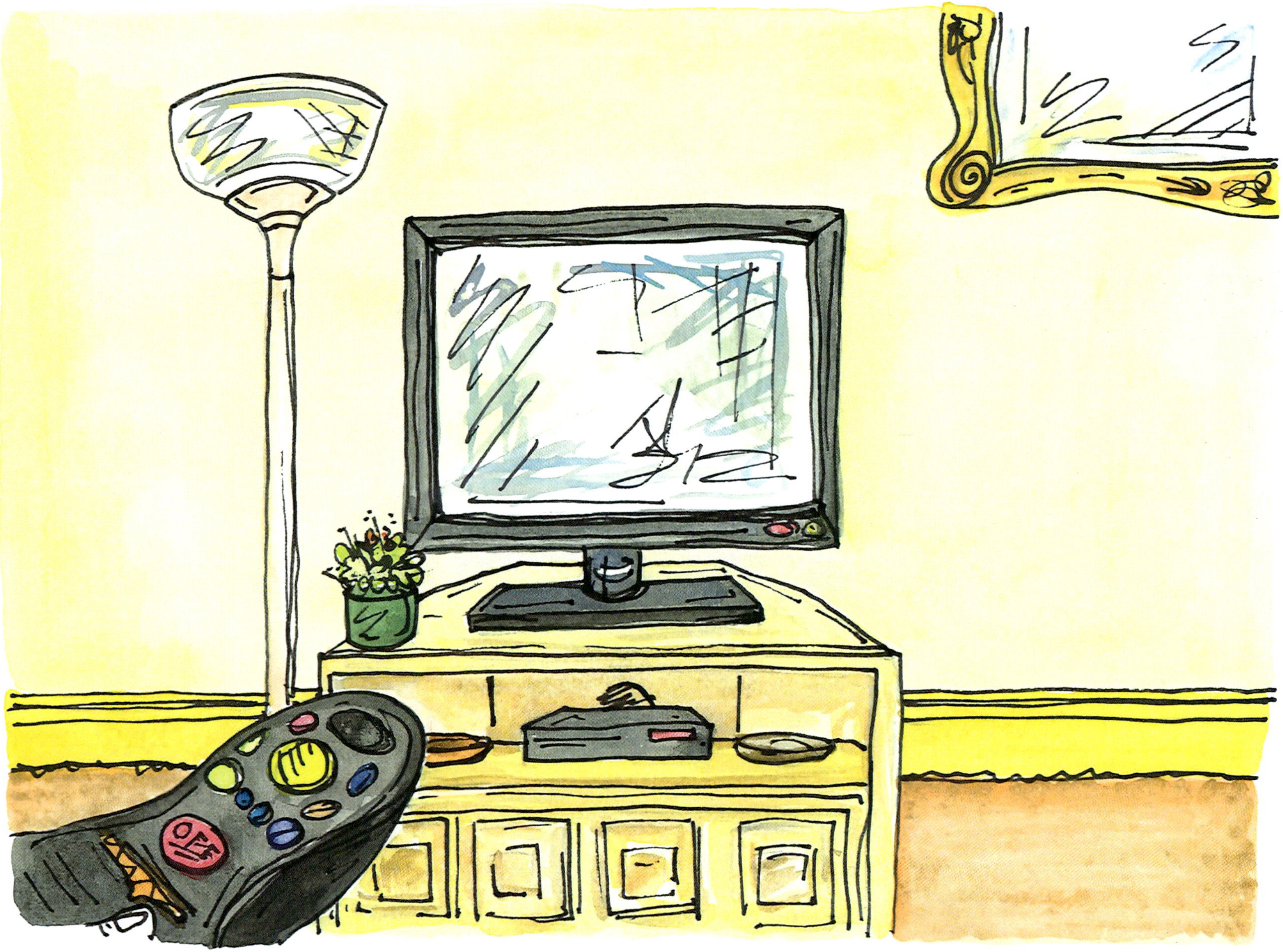

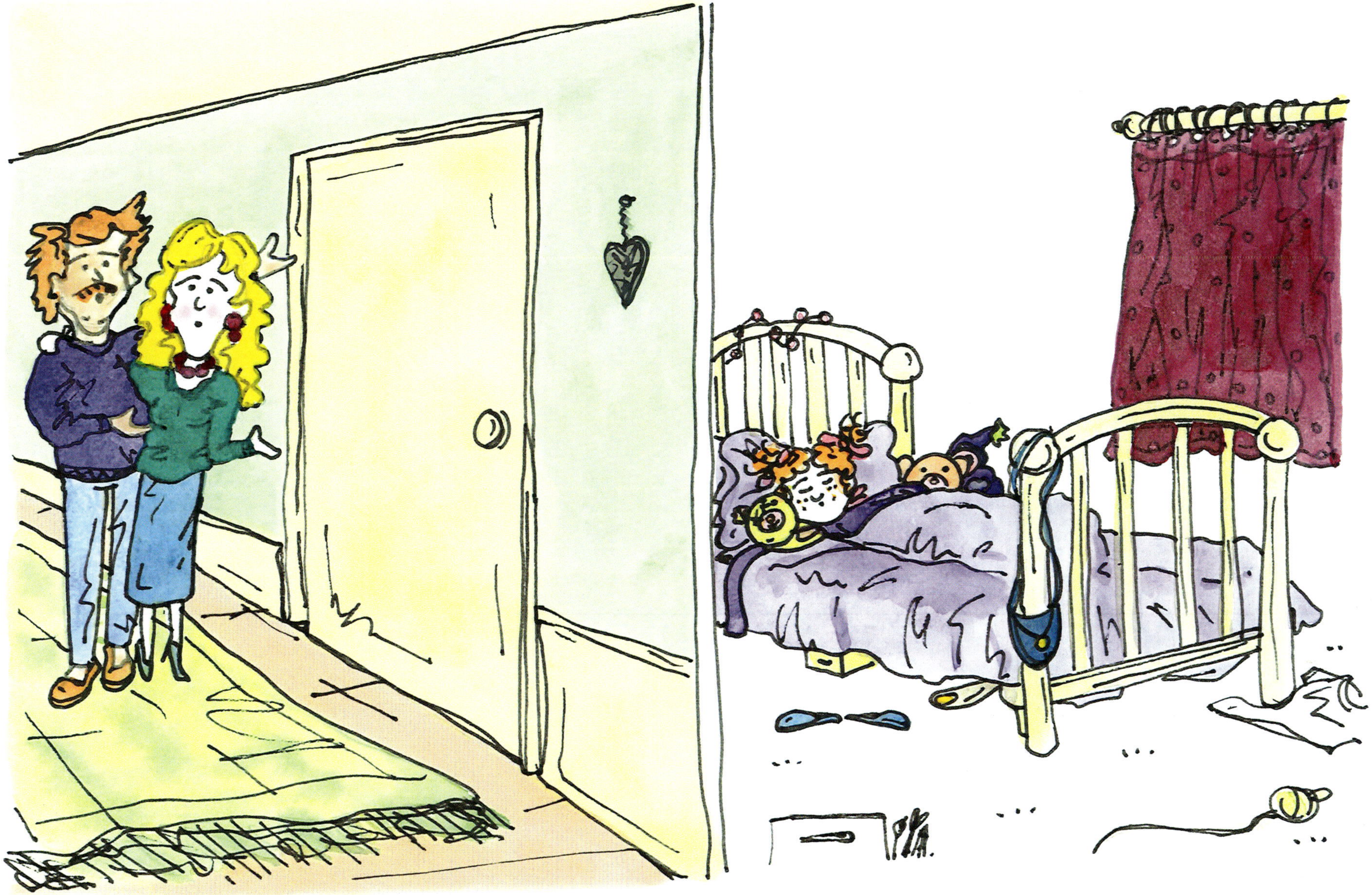

KJ told Lizzie's parents not to run in as soon as Lizzie wakes up in the night. It is very normal for children to shout out or make noises in their sleep.

It does not always mean they are waking up.

Now Lizzie has learnt how healthy it is to fall asleep in her own bed, whilst chatting to herself!

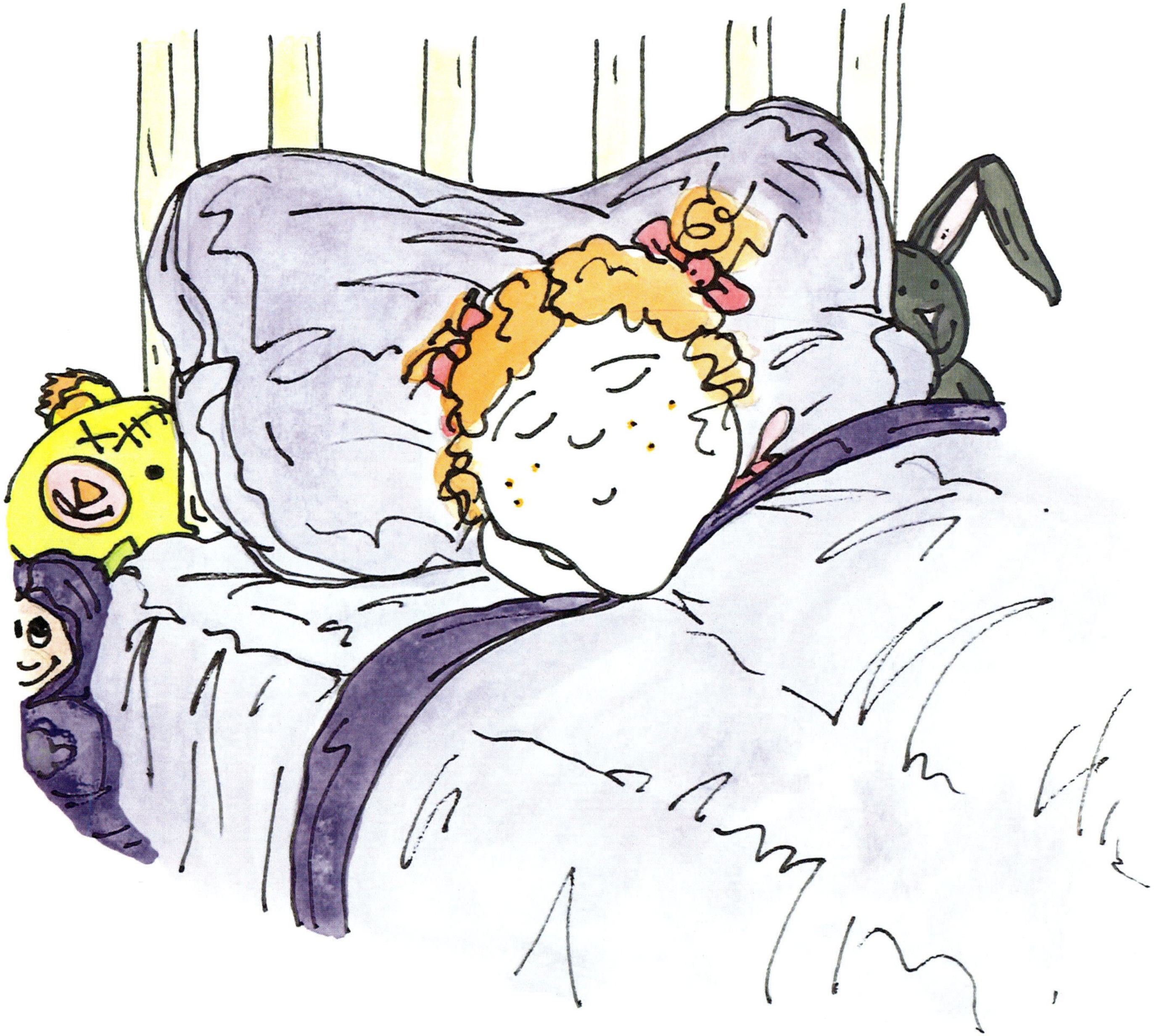

Now all her family have a lovely new routine for bedtime....

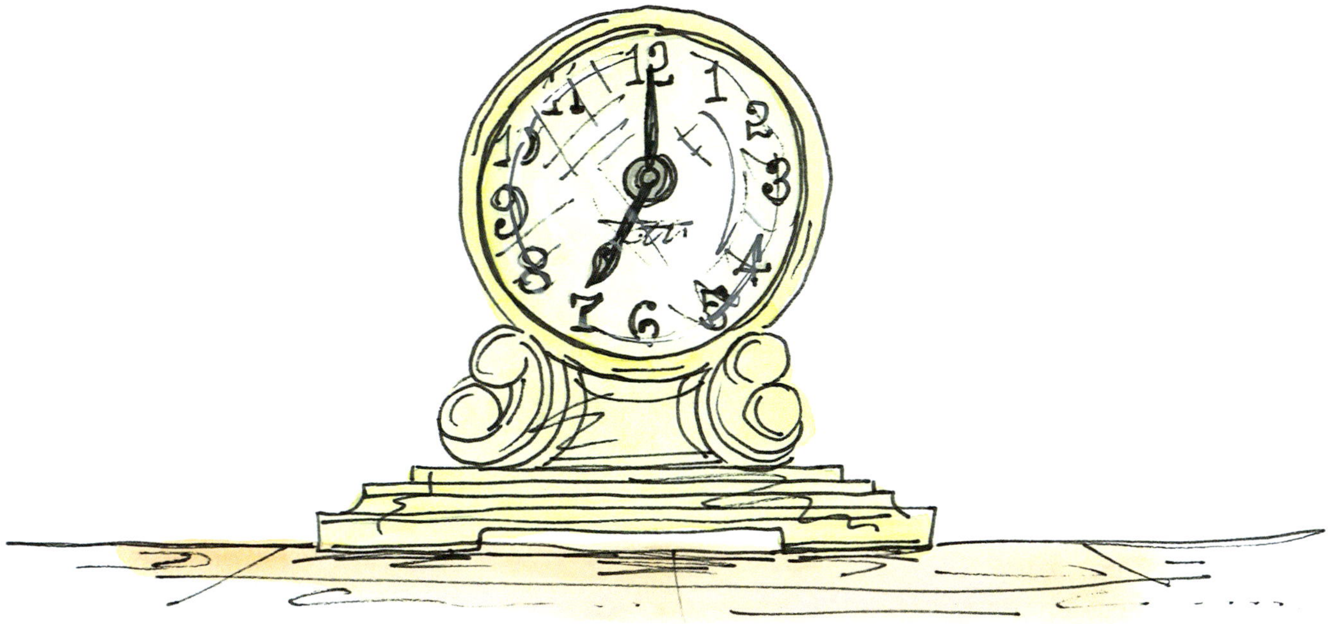

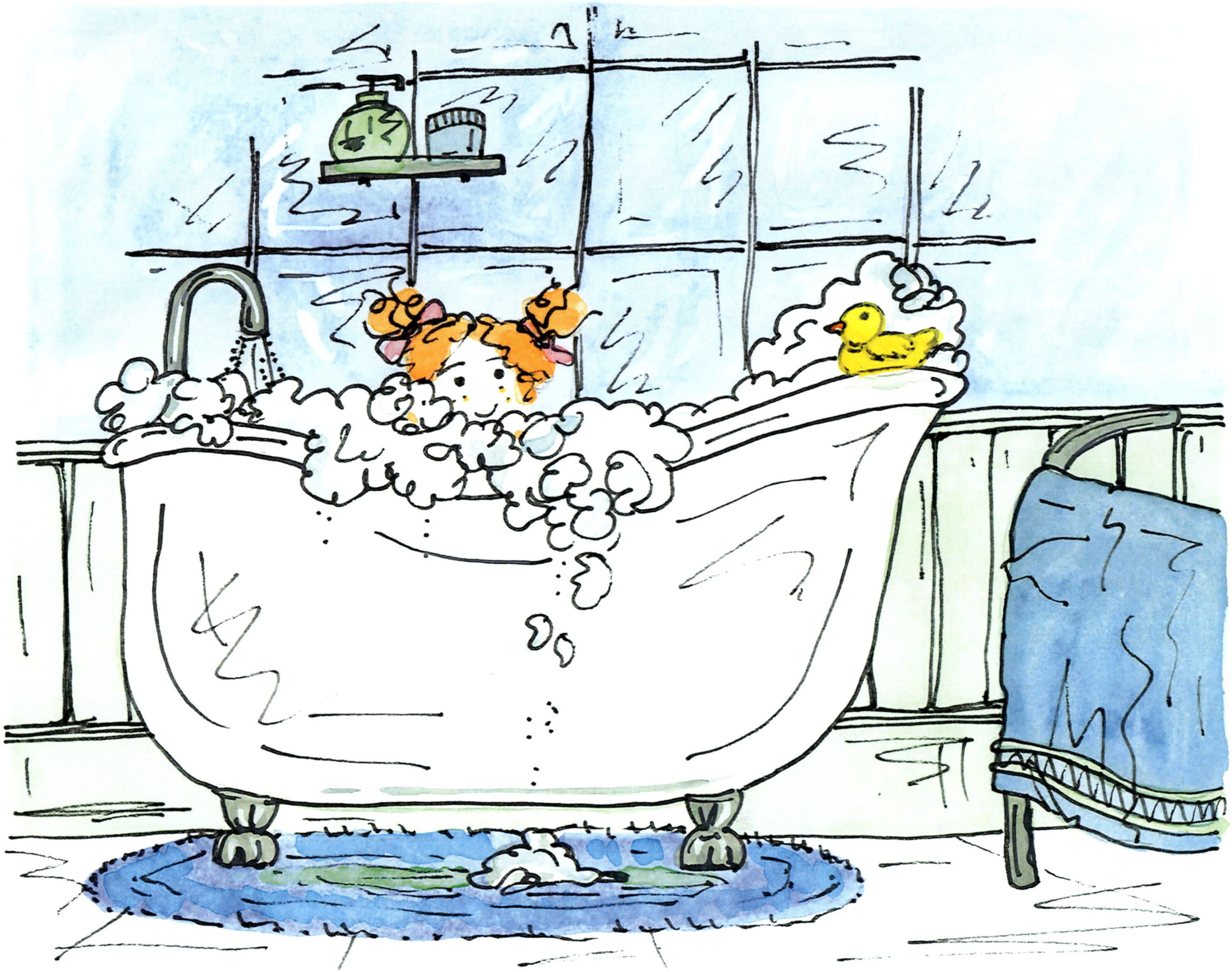

Lizzie has a bath,

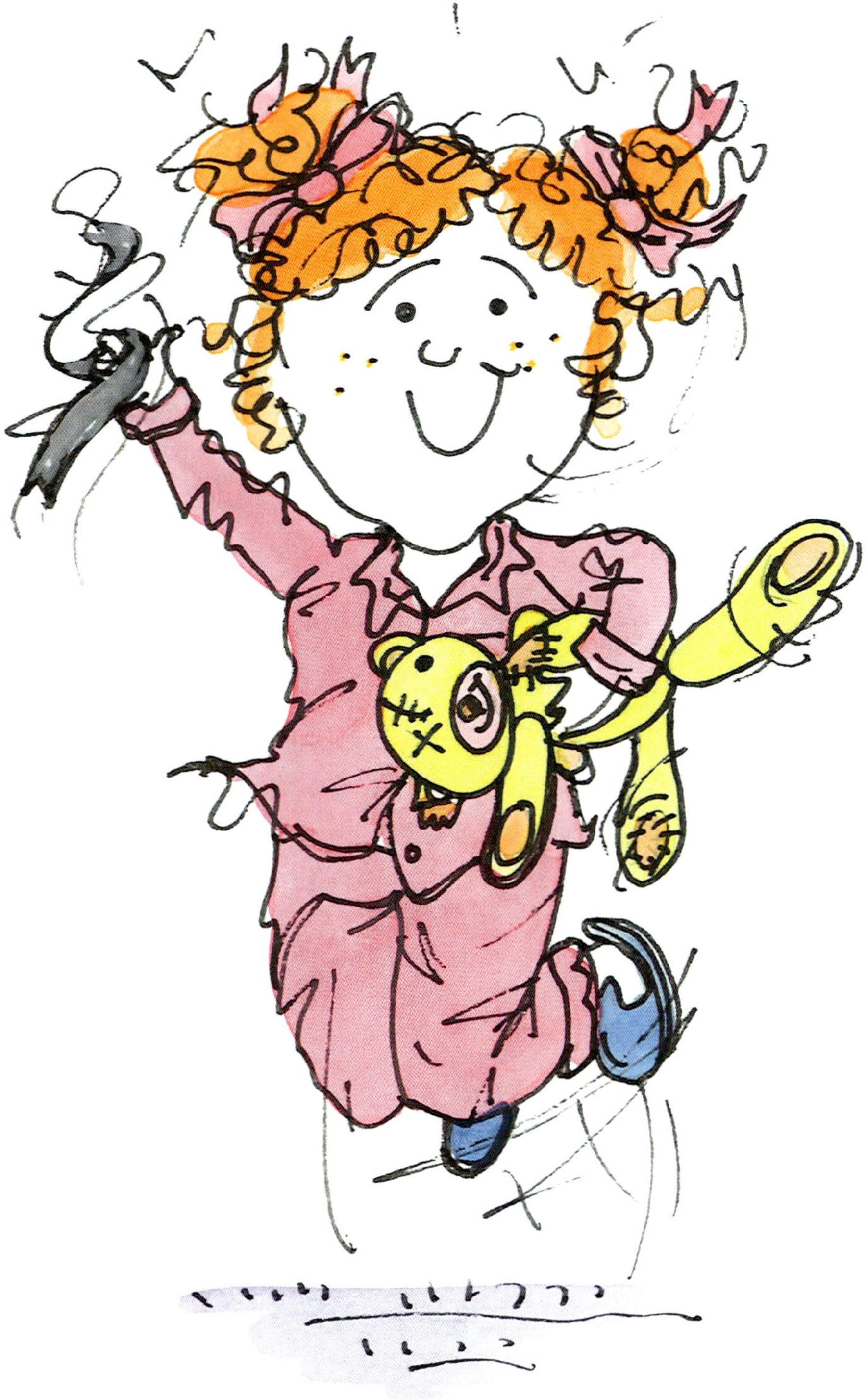

she puts her comfy, cosy pyjamas on
and her parents read her a story or two.

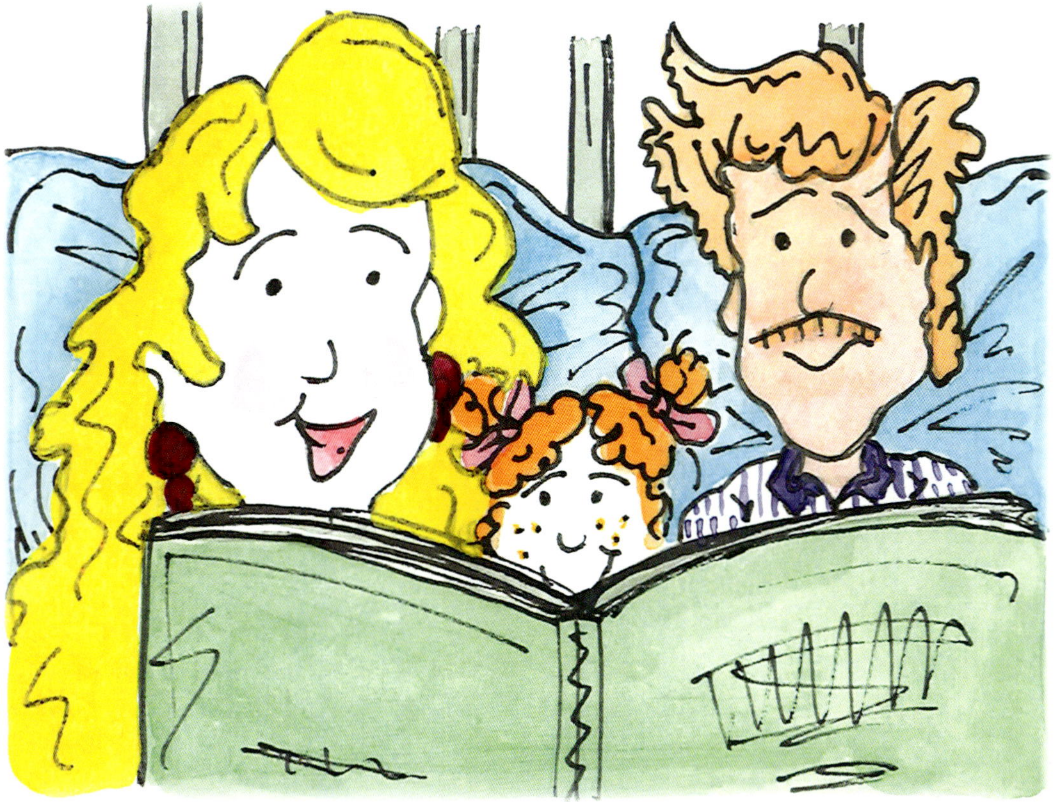

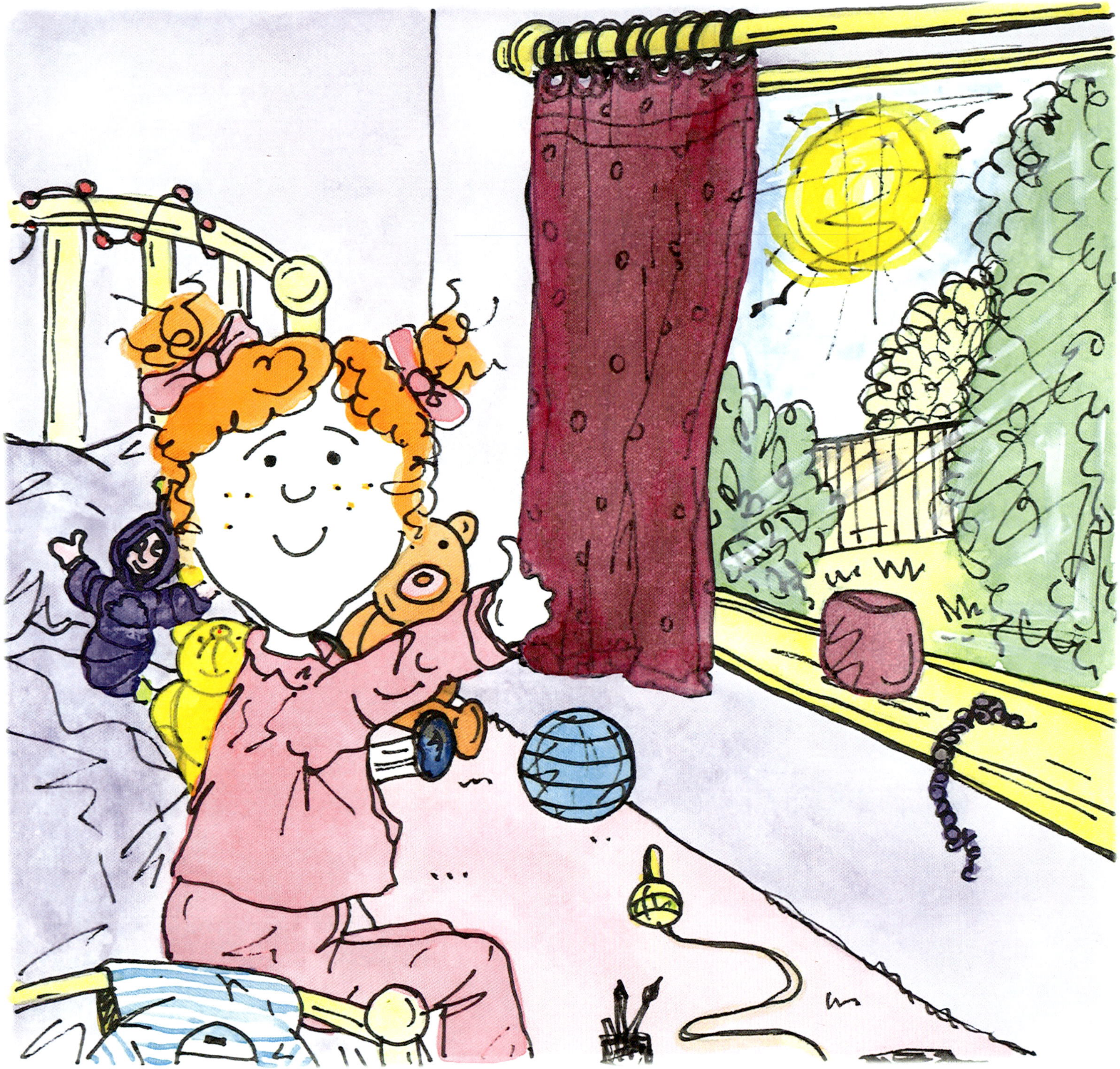

She is now a big girl
and sleeps in her
own bed.

She sleeps all night
until the sun comes up.

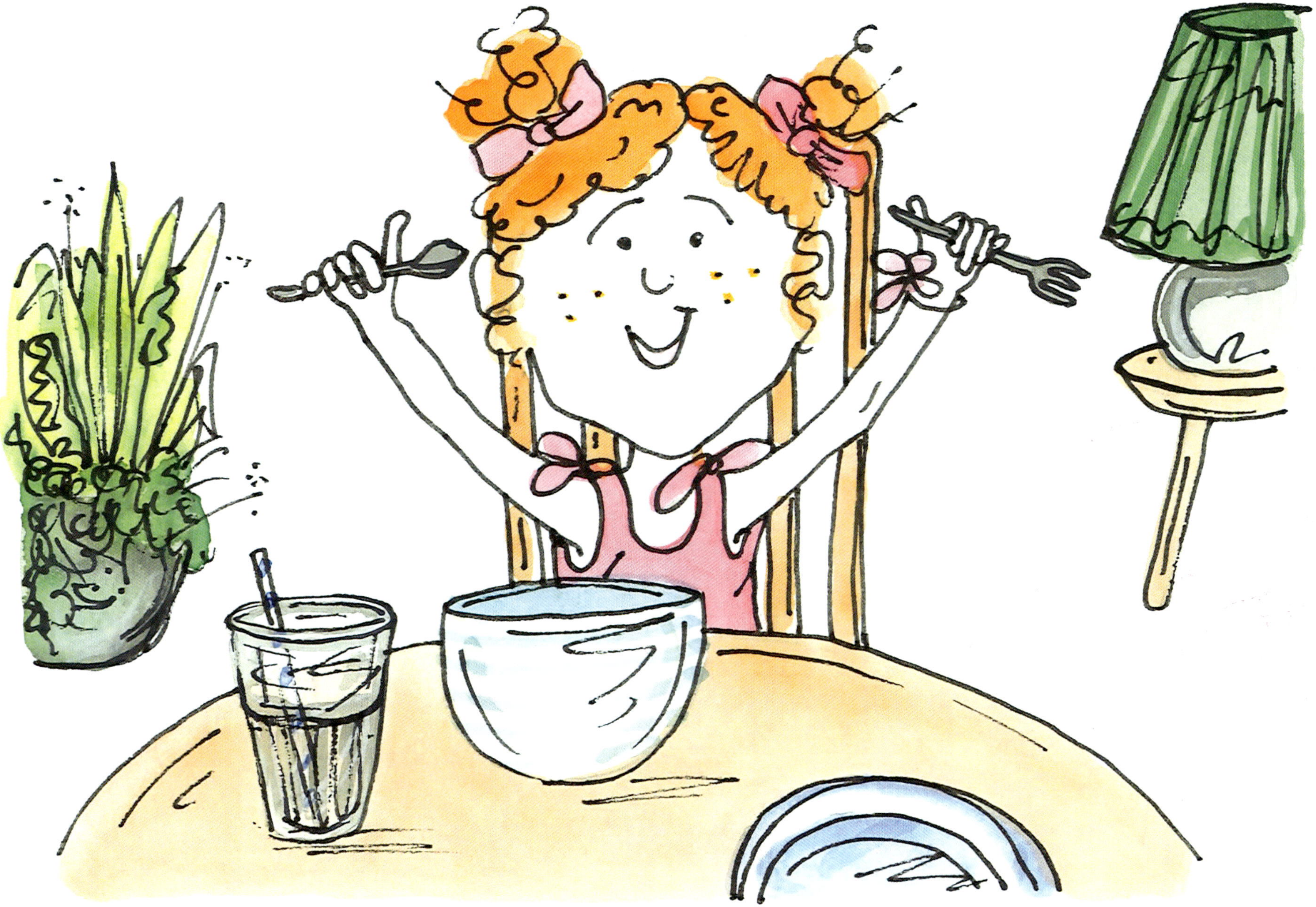

Most of all - she is no longer tired and grumpy and she always finishes her meals.

What a good girl Lizzie is!

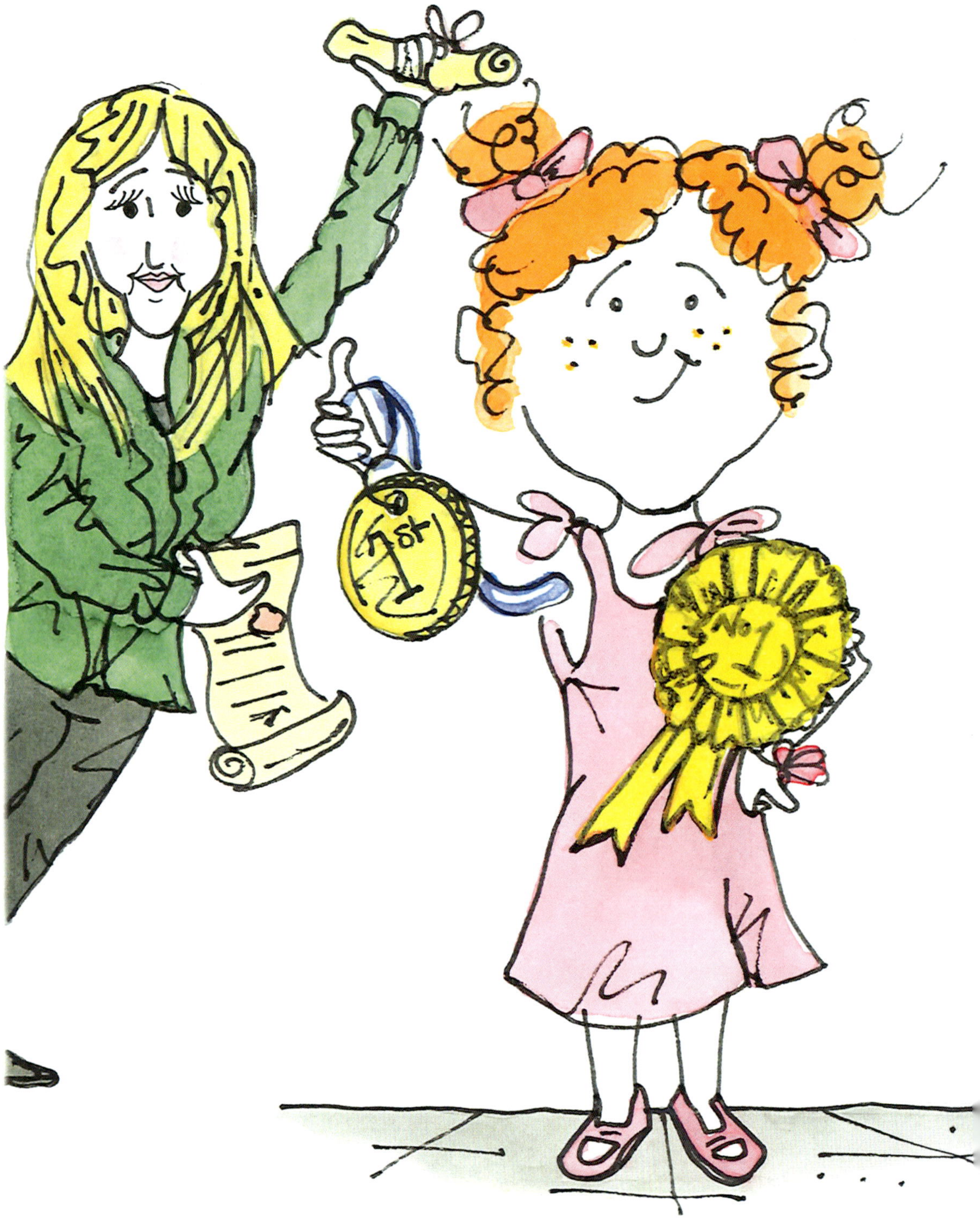

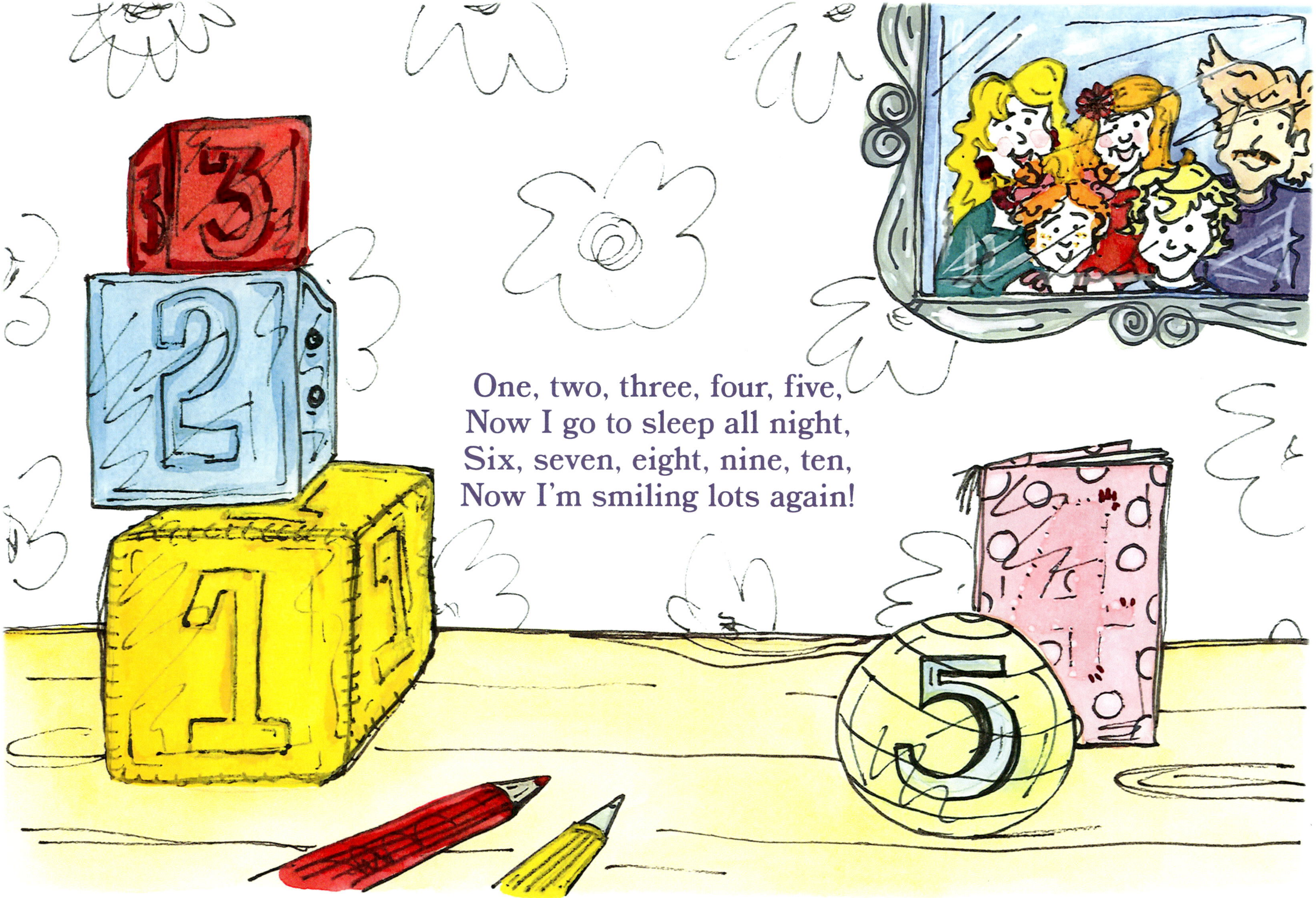

One, two, three, four, five,
Now I go to sleep all night,
Six, seven, eight, nine, ten,
Now I'm smiling lots again!

Instagram: @theinternationalbabywhisperer

Facebook: facebook.com/theinternationalbabywhisperer

Email: hello@theinternationalbabywhisperer.com

Tel: 07522 482873